Why Does My Child Suddenly Hate Me?

Understanding Why Adult Children Suddenly Estrange From Parents

Mez Dawson

© **Copyright 2025 - All rights reserved.**

The content contained within this book may not be reproduced, duplicated or transmitted without direct written permission from the author or the publisher.

Under no circumstances will any blame or legal responsibility be held against the publisher, or author, for any damages, reparation, or monetary loss due to the information contained within this book, either directly or indirectly.

Legal Notice:

This book is copyright protected. It is only for personal use. You cannot amend, distribute, sell, use, quote or paraphrase any part, or the content within this book, without the consent of the author or publisher.

Disclaimer Notice:

Please note the information contained within this document is for educational and entertainment purposes only. All effort has been executed to present accurate, up to date, reliable, complete information. No warranties of any kind are declared or implied. Readers acknowledge that the author is not engaged in the rendering of legal, financial, medical or professional advice. The content within this book has been derived from various sources. Please consult a licensed professional before attempting any techniques outlined in this book.

By reading this document, the reader agrees that under no circumstances is the author responsible for any losses, direct or indirect, that are incurred as a result of the use of the information contained within this document, including, but not limited to, errors, omissions, or inaccuracies.

Table of Contents

TRIGGER WARNING 1

INTRODUCTION 2
    REASONS WHY ADULT CHILDREN TURN AWAY 3
    WHY READ THIS BOOK? 5

CHAPTER 1: UNDERSTANDING THE CAUSES OF ESTRANGEMENT 6
    SOCIETAL INFLUENCES AND MEDIA IMPACT 8
        How Society Has Changed 8
        The Role of Media 9
    PERSONAL CIRCUMSTANCES AND MENTAL HEALTH ISSUES 10
        Individual Trauma 11
        Mental Health Struggles 11
        Life Transitions 11
        Substance Abuse 12
    HOW ABOUT NARCISSISM? 12
    BRINGING IT ALL TOGETHER 14

CHAPTER 2: PARENTS' PERSPECTIVE AND EMOTIONAL CHALLENGES 15
    COPING WITH FALSE ACCUSATIONS AND DEFAMATION 16
        Seek Advice 17
        Write Your Truth 18
        Surround Yourself With Empowering People 18
    MAINTAINING MENTAL WELL-BEING THROUGH GRIEF 19
        Get Moving to Move On 20
        Express Yourself Through Art 20
        Get Professional Help 20
        Build a Fulfilling Routine 21
    CONCLUDING THOUGHTS 21

CHAPTER 3: NAVIGATING THE COMPLEXITIES OF RECONCILIATION 23
    EFFECTIVE COMMUNICATION STRATEGIES 24
        Active Listening 24
        Non-Confrontational Language 24
        Clear Boundaries 25
        Follow-Up Conversations 25
    THE IMPORTANCE OF SELF-REFLECTION 25

- Seeking Professional Help 26
  - Mediation 27
  - Find the Right Professional 27
  - A Two-Side Commitment 28
- Final Insights 28

CHAPTER 4: SUPPORTING YOUR CHILD FROM A DISTANCE 30

- Reaching Out to Your Estranged Child 32
- Understanding Their Perspective and Needs 34
  - Revisiting the Importance of Active Listening 34
  - Honoring Boundaries 35
  - Recognizing and Understanding Triggers 35
- Balancing Support Without Overstepping Boundaries 36
  - Set Norms 36
  - Be Available, Don't Impose Your Help 37
  - Assess Yourself 37
- Concluding Thoughts 38

CHAPTER 5: STAYING RESILIENT AND HOPEFUL 39

- Building a Support Network 39
  - Support Groups 40
  - Online Communities 40
  - Friends You Trust 40
- Exploring Self-Help Strategies and Resources 41
  - Mindfulness 41
  - Keep a Journal 42
  - Take Up a Hobby 42
  - Read 42
- Insights and Implications 43

CONCLUSION 44

REFERENCES 47

Trigger Warning

This book deals with sensitive topics such as

- sexual assault/abuse
- prejudice/discrimination
- child abuse

Introduction

Sometimes, when I'm alone at night in such a big house, I can still hear my children's voices. I don't understand what went wrong. Why did I lose them?

Estrangement from an adult child can feel like an unfathomable whirlwind of emotions leaving parents adrift and longing for the comfort of their family's presence. As I sat alone in the quiet of my living room, the absence of my child's laughter echoed like a haunting melody, reminding me of the days when family meant everything. The silence was more than just a lack of sound; it was a constant reminder of a relationship that had once been plentiful and full of life but now seemed shattered beyond repair. For many parents, this emotional weight is both a personal burden and an unspoken taboo, making it difficult to articulate the depth of their pain.

For those who have never experienced estrangement, it might be easy to simplify or even dismiss these feelings. Yet, as we embark on this narrative journey together, it's crucial to acknowledge the deep emotional landscape in which estranged parents find themselves. This book will become a companion through that landscape, providing understanding, support, and practical advice as you navigate these turbulent times.

Reasons Why Adult Children Turn Away

We often assume that family bonds are unbreakable, yet many find themselves at a crossroads where estrangement feels like the only option, driven by unrecognized grief, unmet needs, or toxic circumstances. These realities form the backdrop of our exploration, painting a nuanced picture of why estrangement occurs and what it means for those involved.

Family estrangement is a complex issue with a kaleidoscope of contributing factors, such as

- mental health struggles, those silent battles fought within the confines of one's mind that often spill over into relationships.

- societal changes, which create a chasm between generations, leading to misunderstandings that become insurmountable barriers.

- moments when communication breaks down entirely, leaving behind a void where love and warmth once resided.

In the world of estrangement, parents frequently find themselves grappling with feelings of loss, confusion, and helplessness. In the stillness of the night, a parent might reflect on the myriad of accusations hurled their way, each one like a dagger piercing their heart. The weight of false narratives becomes overwhelming, making them question every decision they made during their child's upbringing. Were they too strict? Too lenient? Did they fail to see the signs of distress early enough? These questions circle endlessly, adding to the already heavy burden of emotional turmoil.

But amid this darkness, there exists a glimmer of hope. Imagine a moment when the silence of estrangement is broken; the tentative bleat of a message filled with curiosity has the power to ignite healing and understanding. While resolution may seem distant and daunting, it is not impossible. It requires patience, compassion, and a willingness to embrace vulnerability, both from the parents' side and, ideally, from the estranged children as well. Understanding must come before reconciliation, and communication is the bridge that can lead both parties back to common ground.

Why Read This Book?

This book seeks to guide you on that journey toward resolution, offering insights and strategies gleaned from multiple perspectives, including the voices of mental health professionals and counselors who specialize in family dynamics. Whether you're a parent desperately seeking answers or a mental health professional looking to support your clients more effectively, this narrative provides a beacon of hope, illuminating paths that others have taken and showing that healing is possible, even if it seems improbable at first glance.

As we delve deeper into the chapters ahead, remember that you are not alone in this experience. Countless others share similar stories, each marked by its own unique set of challenges and triumphs. The path to reconciliation is seldom straightforward, but with unwavering effort and empathy, it can lead to newfound connections and stronger family ties. Let us venture together into this path, armed with understanding and an open heart, as we explore ways to mend the broken bonds of family estrangement.

Chapter 1:

Understanding the Causes of Estrangement

Albert had been a single father for over three decades. Throughout those years, his relationship with Mike, his only son, oscillated between warmth and distance. This dynamic changed abruptly when Mike got married, leading to a sudden silence on his end. Albert found himself grappling with confusion and regret, questioning the choices he had made in their past.

After Mike's marriage, the phone calls that once flowed freely became infrequent and ultimately ceased. Albert was left pondering how their bond, once filled with laughter and shared experiences, had degenerated into a quiet void. This shift made him reflect on their history, searching for answers in the memories they had created together. What had he overlooked during the tumultuous years of parenthood that might have altered the course of their relationship?

The first step to finding a resolution for estrangement is by understanding its causes. As societal values shift and cultural norms evolve, these changes profoundly impact how adult children view their relationships with parents. The very fabric of what constitutes a family is knit from threads that are being pulled in new directions, influenced by individualism and diverse family structures. These shifts can leave parents feeling adrift, struggling to reconcile the expectations they grew up with and those held by their children. It's a journey of rediscovery where the ways we communicate and connect are continually transforming, often in ways that deepen the divide rather than bridge it. In this evolving landscape, the voices and choices of adult children reflect broader narratives of personal autonomy and self-fulfillment, challenging traditional roles and loyalties.

In this chapter, we'll explore some reasons adult children may distance themselves from their parents, offering insights that go beyond surface-level interpretations. From societal influences and media representations to the complex interplay between personal circumstances, mental health challenges, and life transitions, we'll assess how these factors contribute significantly to why some individuals choose separation as a means to cope with unresolved trauma or navigate new phases of their lives.

Societal Influences and Media Impact

You may feel isolated while navigating estrangement, but you are far from being alone. Numbers don't lie: According to a study from Cornell University, 27% of adults in the US have cut ties with at least one family member (Dean, 2020). Why is this phenomenon suddenly so common?

In recent years, a shift in societal values has begun to reshape how adult children perceive their relationships with their parents. The concept of family is no longer bound by traditional roles and expectations. Instead, it is constantly evolving, influenced by a myriad of factors, including cultural shifts. These changes have challenged conventional ideas about family dynamics, leaving many parents grasping for understanding as they navigate an unfamiliar landscape.

How Society Has Changed

One major cultural shift involves the increasing emphasis on individualism over familial obligation. In a world that often prioritizes personal happiness and self-fulfillment, adult children may feel less compelled to maintain relationships that they perceive as unsatisfying or emotionally draining. According to psychologist Dr. Joshua Coleman, we're living in a less family-oriented culture than in the past: "Our young adults value happiness and autonomy. If the relationship with the parent is stressful, they will rather walk away" (Henkelman, 2024). This perspective can be jarring for parents who were raised with a strong sense of duty toward family.

Moreover, the rise of diverse family structures—single-parent homes, blended families, and chosen families—has broadened what it means to belong to a family unit. Children growing up in these varied environments might adopt new norms that diverge significantly from those of their parents' generation.

Finally, peer pressure cannot be overlooked when examining the reasons behind family estrangement. Just as in adolescence, adults are not immune to the influence of their peers. Friends and colleagues can impact one's thoughts and actions regarding family through shared beliefs and conversations. When peers share similar experiences or frustrations about parental relationships, this can create a sense of solidarity that validates an individual's decision to distance themselves. Group dynamics can further reinforce these beliefs, making it challenging for individuals to see other perspectives or reconsider their choices.

The Role of Media

As society continues to evolve, so does its communication landscape. Let's see how new and traditional media may influence estrangement.

Social Media

Social media platforms have become powerful tools in shaping opinions and experiences, offering spaces where individuals can find communities that resonate with their perspectives. For adult children, these online interactions can reinforce their views on family relationships, sometimes validating feelings of estrangement.

Curated content on social media often presents idealized versions of family life, which can lead to unrealistic expectations and dissatisfaction. Additionally, encountering stories of others who have distanced themselves from their families can make such decisions seem more acceptable or common, further influencing one's own choices.

Mainstream Media

Parallel to social media's impact, the portrayal of family dynamics in mainstream media also plays a significant role in shaping perceptions. Films, television shows, and books frequently simplify complex familial issues and present them in easily digestible narratives.

While this can make for compelling storytelling, it can also distort reality, leading audiences to misunderstand the intricacies of real-life family relationships. For instance, media representations of estranged family members often focus on dramatic reconciliations or clear-cut villains, neglecting the nuanced emotions and situations involved in these relationships. This oversimplification could contribute to skewed societal attitudes, leading some to believe that estrangement is either easily resolvable or justified in binary terms.

These societal influences collectively contribute to a broader understanding of why adult children might choose estrangement as a path. Parents navigating these waters need to recognize that today's world presents children with new paradigms and norms that might conflict with their upbringing.

Understanding the impact of cultural shifts, social media, media representation, and peer pressure can offer insight into the thinking of estranged children. It can also provide a starting point for empathy, encouraging parents to engage in open dialogues that honor both generations' experiences and perspectives.

Personal Circumstances and Mental Health Issues

Behind the decision to cut off a family member (or several of them), there's always a painful path. As Peg Streep from *Psychology Today* puts it, no functional adult happily decides to become an orphan all of a sudden: "No one estranges from their parents or family of origin as an option of first choice; it is usually a last-ditch effort to put an end to an emotionally untenable situation" (2023). Let's explore the most significant contributors for estrangement.

Individual Trauma

Trauma from childhood can leave deep scars that influence one's ability to maintain healthy relationships later in life. Experiences such as neglect, abuse, or a lack of emotional support during formative years can develop into coping mechanisms that lead to distancing oneself from others, including family members. The cycle of unresolved trauma may manifest in adulthood as estrangement from parents. Adult children might subconsciously associate their current family dynamics with past painful experiences, prompting them to distance themselves as a way to protect their emotional well-being.

Mental Health Struggles

Conditions like depression and anxiety are known to create barriers to effective communication and relationship-building. When an individual grapples with these mental health challenges, they may find it difficult to express their needs and feelings clearly, leading to misunderstandings and conflicts within the family unit. This disconnect can prompt adult children to seek distance from their parents as a means of managing overwhelming emotions or avoiding conflict altogether. Furthermore, mental health issues can exacerbate feelings of isolation and alienation, further straining familial bonds (Ergenzinger, 2022).

Life Transitions

Major changes such as getting married, having children, or relocating can shift priorities and reconfigure one's social landscape. These transitions may inadvertently lead to neglecting parental relationships as new responsibilities and roles take precedence. For instance, as it happened to Mike in the beginning of this chapter, marriage often introduces a partner's family into the dynamic, altering traditional loyalties and energy allocation. Similarly, becoming a parent typically demands an immense focus on nurturing the next generation, potentially sidelining the previous one.

Substance Abuse

Alcohol or drug misuse can severely strain relationships, often resulting in disappointment and betrayal among family members (Ergenzinger, 2022). When substance abuse is present, trust erodes and communication falters, making reconciliation challenging. Adult children may choose to distance themselves to avoid enabling behavior or experiencing recurrent hurt or frustration associated with addiction. Substance abuse not only impacts interpersonal dynamics but also challenges families with cyclical patterns of recovery and relapse, further complicating reconciliation efforts.

How About Narcissism?

Although it's common to hear that the reason for family estrangement is due to growing up with narcissistic parents, full-blown narcissism isn't as frequent as we'd expect: While many people display some narcissistic traits—such as selfishness, a lack of ability to handle criticism, emotional or verbal abuse, or a lack of empathy—only one percent of the population has narcissistic personality disorder (NPD) (Lis, 2022).

Narcissism is believed to have a genetic component as well as being influenced by certain family dynamics. Therefore, when either parents or adult children feel tempted to label "narcissism" as the reason for estrangement, they should consider assessing their own traits before fully labelling the other person. This takes a lot of introspection, hard work, and courage. Working alongside a professional may help.

However, we mustn't overlook the pain inflicted by narcissistic adult children: While NPD is influenced by genetics, its causes are way more complex. For a start, narcissism usually occurs with other brain and personality disorders, which means its "basis is more than a cut-and-dried scenario where parents are to blame" (McGregor, 2024).

Parents of narcissistic adult children experience guilt and regret (constantly wondering what they could have done differently), and are burdened with the task of dealing with a seemingly endless teenage stage, as described by author Chelsey Cole: "If your adult child is a narcissist, it's like your child never grows up. They're stuck in perpetual adolescence" (Trepany, 2024). However, unlike what happens when adults determinately cut ties with their narcissistic parents, this doesn't work the other way around: Parents often find themselves subjects of emotional, verbal, and financial abuse, but can't set boundaries with their adult children. We'll see more about this topic in the following chapter.

While these personal challenges and mental health issues significantly contribute to estrangement, it's essential to approach each situation with empathy and understanding. Recognizing the multifaceted nature of these issues can empower both parents and adult children to navigate their complex emotions and work toward healing their relationships if they choose. It requires acknowledging past traumas, addressing mental health care, adapting wisely to life changes, and tackling substance abuse head-on.

An open dialogue about these topics can be a good starting point for bridging gaps. Engaging in therapy, either individually or as a family unit, could offer insights and strategies to manage these challenges constructively. Family members should strive for mutual understanding and give each other space to process their unique journeys. Rebuilding strained bonds takes time and patience, and sometimes professional guidance becomes indispensable in fostering healthier connections.

Bringing It All Together

In this chapter, we've delved into various reasons that might lead adult children to distance themselves from their parents, highlighting both societal influences and personal circumstances:

- From the cultural shift toward individualism and the powerful sway of social media to evolving norms within diverse family structures, these factors reshape perceptions of familial ties.

- Media portrayals can sometimes simplify complex issues, while peer pressure reinforces decisions to separate.

- Personal challenges and mental health issues—including narcissistic traits—lie at the heart of many estrangements.

- Childhood trauma, mental health struggles, life transitions, and substance abuse contribute deeply to the decision to distance oneself.

These issues often intertwine, making reconciliation an intricate process. Yet, acknowledging these struggles can empower families to address them constructively, perhaps through therapy or open conversations. Ultimately, the healing journey is personal and requires patience, empathy, and sometimes professional guidance.

As parents and children navigate their unique pathways, understanding remains a vital step toward rebuilding and nurturing familial bonds. Our next chapter will explore your perspective as a parent and the unique emotional challenges you may face.

Chapter 2:

Parents' Perspective and Emotional Challenges

At 52, Sarah, a dedicated single mother, devoted her life to raising her daughter Emily independently. Juggling multiple jobs, she made countless sacrifices to ensure Emily received a top-notch education, always prioritizing her daughter's needs above her own. However, as Emily matured, Sarah became increasingly concerned about her daughter's behavior—Emily displayed a lack of empathy, often manipulating Sarah and craving constant admiration while showing scant gratitude. She attributed every challenge in her life to her mother's shortcomings. As an adult, Emily grew more self-centered and demanding, relying on Sarah for financial support, validation, and emotional comfort, yet offering nothing in return.

No matter how hard Sarah tried and despite her unwavering love, Emily treated her with contempt. She belittled her mother's struggles, dismissed every single one of her sacrifices, and only reached out when she needed financial help. Whenever Sarah set a boundary, Emily would accuse her of being selfish or dramatic.

Emily often rewrote history, making Sarah question her own experiences. If Sarah recalled a time she made a sacrifice for Emily, Emily dismissed it: "You never did anything special for me. Other parents did way more for their kids." She would also blame Sarah for any struggles in her life: "Maybe if you had been a better mother, it wouldn't be so difficult for me now." Emily kept twisting the situation until Sarah felt guilty for even trying to stand up for herself: "You're toxic. I need to cut you out of my life for my mental health."

When Sarah finally confronted Emily about the emotional abuse by refusing to give her more money, Emily exploded in rage. "You're the problem, not me," she snapped before cutting off contact completely, leaving Sarah heartbroken and confused.

Like Sarah, parents during estrangement are often riddled with feelings of confusion and loneliness. The weight of not having contact with their adult children can manifest in various emotional challenges that are difficult to navigate alone. For many parents, this separation brings an unexpected shift in their roles and responsibilities, leaving them grappling with the loss of connection that once defined their family dynamic.

Sarah now mourns the daughter she nurtured, struggling with feelings of failure and uncertainty about her parenting. As we can see, it is not only the absence of physical presence that impacts these parents but also the haunting silence that follows. In this chapter, we'll delve into these intricate emotions and shed light on the multifaceted aspects that make estrangement so uniquely painful. Additionally, we'll also go through practical strategies for maintaining mental well-being through grief. Hopefully, you'll find both validation and guidance to navigating the rocky terrain of estrangement.

Coping With False Accusations and Defamation

While you are far from being the only parent estranged from their adult children, the topic remains somehow a taboo. Cultural shifts and societal pressure, as seen in Chapter 1, have made things easier for adult children speaking up—and blaming their parents for every problem—but certainly, not the other way around. Parents often find themselves harshly judged by media and professionals who are too fast to raise their accusatory fingers.

Let's go back to Sarah's example. Experiencing estrangement from a narcissistic child can be one of the deepest wounds a parent endures. Society often looks to blame the parent, assuming there must have been a misstep. However, narcissistic individuals distort reality, cast themselves as victims, and evade responsibility. Ultimately, a mother may find herself left with no choice but to grieve the lost relationship and seek solace in the love she offered, while holding onto the hope of a future reconciliation.

In the challenging landscape of estrangement, navigating through false accusations can weigh heavily on parents. These baseless claims not only tarnish reputations but also inflict emotional distress that leaves many grappling with feelings of isolation and self-doubt. It's important to understand the psychological impact these accusations have. When faced with unfounded allegations, parents might begin questioning their own actions and identities, leading to a profound sense of loneliness. This mental turmoil is often exacerbated by the erosion of trust in familial relationships, leaving parents feeling alienated from their adult children.

Developing resilience amidst character defamation becomes crucial in managing such emotional upheaval. Parents need to arm themselves with coping strategies that foster emotional strength. Let's see some strategies you can start implementing.

Seek Advice

Your adult child may spread rumors regarding, for instance, your behavior or mental health, which can affect your reputation or even take a toll on your other personal or professional relationships. Tackling public misconceptions requires an understanding that while perceptions may vary, one's truth remains steadfast.

Seeking legal or professional advice stands out as a pivotal step in combating severe defamation. Legal counsel can provide guidance on how best to navigate potential disputes, whereas mental health professionals can offer emotional support and techniques for managing stress and anxiety related to false accusations (*Uncovering the Nightmare*, 2023).

Write Your Truth

Personal reflection plays a vital role in countering the damaging effects of false narratives. Keeping a journal can be an effective tool for parents to articulate their feelings and confront emotions head-on.

This is what eventually helped Sarah recognize narcissistic traits in her daughter Emily: After every painful encounter with her daughter, Sarah wrote down specific, harmful remarks she got. For example, Emily expects Sarah to provide financial help without gratitude. When Sarah hesitates to loan her money, this is how Emily responds: "Wow, after everything I've done for you, you can't even help your own daughter?" (despite Emily rarely helping Sarah in return). Or recently, when Sarah underwent surgery and reached out to Emily for support only to receive a dismissive response: "I'm really busy right now. I can't deal with your drama."

As painful as it is to see these statements on paper, they help Sarah realize the truth. Writing about one's experiences not only helps process complex emotions but also aids in identifying and challenging negative thoughts that perpetuate self-doubt. This reflective practice offers clarity and helps individuals reclaim control over their narrative.

Moreover, regular journaling provides a safe space for introspection, allowing parents to track personal growth and resilience over time, reinforcing their journey of healing and empowerment. We'll see more about this in Chapter 5.

Surround Yourself With Empowering People

Building a supportive community is another crucial component in managing the emotional fallout of false accusations. Surrounding oneself with trusted family members and friends who believe in their innocence offers significant solace during such trying times. Sharing experiences within this circle not only alleviates feelings of alienation but also reinforces a network of emotional support.

Engaging in community groups or forums where similar stories are exchanged can further build connections and instill a sense of belonging. For instance, attending support groups or participating in online forums dedicated to wrongful accusations can offer new perspectives and shared empathy, which are instrumental in the healing process (Brooks & Greenberg, 2020).

Maintaining Mental Well-Being Through Grief

The emotional challenges faced by parents experiencing estrangement can be profoundly distressing. Understanding mental health during these periods is crucial for navigating the complex emotional landscape. While everyone can show sympathy and support to grieving parents who lost an adult child due to a premature death, in the case of family estrangement, the public displays of support are often limited by bias and misconceptions. However, recognizing estrangement as a form of loss allows parents to validate their emotions and embark on a healing journey.

Estrangement triggers a grieving process similar to other forms of loss, such as divorce or death, though it is often accompanied by unique complexities. This type of grief can include feelings of rejection, confusion, and prolonged sadness. However, acknowledging these emotions as a natural response to estrangement can help parents understand that their reactions are normal and part of a broader process of healing (Burford, 2024).

While we may feel tempted to hide negative feelings such as guilt, regret, or even anger toward our adult children, embracing emotions rather than suppressing them encourages healing. You don't grieve the loss of your child's life, but you still grieve the loss of *a* life—the family life you once had or longed for. The feeling is normal and valid. Several strategies can help manage this grief effectively. Let's discuss them.

Get Moving to Move On

Physical activities serve as a constructive outlet for pent-up emotions and stress. Whether it's a structured exercise routine, like jogging or yoga, or engaging in an energetic activity such as dancing, movement can help release endorphins and improve overall mood. Consistently incorporating physical activity into one's life not only aids in managing grief but also enhances physical health, which in turn supports mental well-being.

Express Yourself Through Art

Painting, singing, sculpting, or writing provide therapeutic benefits for emotional release. Creating something tangible from intangible emotions helps articulate feelings and can lead to insights that might otherwise remain hidden. By externalizing emotions through creativity, parents may find a renewed sense of purpose.

Get Professional Help

Exploring counseling options is another vital strategy in managing the emotional fallout of estrangement. Therapists can offer tools and frameworks to process complex emotions, aiding parents in navigating the intricate dynamics of estranged relationships. Cognitive behavioral therapy (CBT) or trauma-informed approaches may be particularly beneficial when dealing with complicated or entrenched grief (*Coping With Family Estrangement*, 2024).

How about group therapy? Being part of a group where others share similar experiences allows parents to feel less isolated and more supported. Sharing personal stories and hearing others' journeys can be enlightening and reassuring, demonstrating that they are not alone in their struggles, while also fostering the exchange of practical advice and coping mechanisms that have worked for others.

Build a Fulfilling Routine

Establishing a consistent routine is crucial for fostering stability and reviving one's spirit. A routine offers a reassuring framework amid disorder, allowing parents to reclaim control over their lives. Regular meal times, sleep schedules, and daily tasks create a sense of order. Equally vital is integrating self-care into these routines. Activities such as enjoying a warm bath, immersing in a captivating book, or engaging in a beloved hobby enhance emotional strength.

To cultivate healthy habits, reserving time for personal interests is essential for rejuvenation. Whether it's gardening, playing an instrument, or painting, these activities help redirect focus from challenges toward personal development and satisfaction. Engaging in hobbies can also lead to new social connections, broadening support networks beyond immediate circles.

Concluding Thoughts

Navigating the emotional journey of estrangement is a deep challenge for parents, marked by feelings of grief and loss similar to other life-changing events. Throughout this chapter, we have discussed the complex emotions that arise when facing false accusations and defamation within familial relationships. By exploring practical strategies, parents are encouraged to find their path to resilience and empowerment.

Understanding that experiencing estrangement triggers a grieving process helps validate the emotions involved. Acknowledging feelings of rejection and sadness is a natural response in your healing journey. We've noticed the importance of healthy coping mechanisms such as

- mindfulness practices
- physical activities
- counseling

- a healthy routine

By embracing these tools, you are equipped to not only confront the challenges of estrangement but also rediscover hope and personal fulfillment beyond your current struggles. Besides, you'll open the possibility of a reconciliation—the topic for our next chapter.

Chapter 3:

Navigating the Complexities of Reconciliation

Strengthening yourself and embracing life's possibilities when struggling with family estrangement is certainly a must. However, a parent will never stop loving their child. If there's a chance to bring them back into your life, you'll probably want to explore it.

But you must know that rebuilding relationships with estranged children involves navigating a labyrinth of emotional complexities and communication hurdles. Reconciliation is an intricate process that requires patience, understanding, and effective strategies to bridge gaps. Many parents find themselves yearning for a reconciliation that not only mends the past but also builds a stronger foundation for future interactions.

So is reconciliation possible? It is! Is it easy? Most certainly not! This journey often begins with acknowledging the depth of estrangement and the specific challenges it brings, setting the stage for meaningful dialogue and growth. As families embark on this sensitive path, nothing is as important as communicating effectively, guiding every step toward healing.

In this chapter, we dive into the vital art of communication as a core element in the reconciliation process. You'll discover practical tools designed to foster open and honest dialogue between parents and their adult children. Additionally, we'll offer insights into establishing clear boundaries that respect each party's needs and emotions.

Effective Communication Strategies

Any attempt of reconciliation with an estranged adult child can be an emotionally challenging journey for parents seeking to rebuild relationships. The art of communication, where opening lines of dialogue can encourage understanding and healing, provides parents with effective tools to engage in meaningful conversations. Let's examine the elements of such a crucial component of any healthy relationship.

Active Listening

This foundational skill creates a safe space for both parties involved by validating emotions and showing a genuine desire to understand. Whenever you and your estranged child try to talk, do you listen with a response already in mind? Or do you truly try to put yourself into their shoes? For example, if a child shares feelings of past hurt, a parent might say, "I hear you, and I understand how that must have felt," rather than immediately offering solutions or dismissals. Acknowledging pain validates experiences and lays the groundwork for trust, signaling that their voice matters. We'll see more about this in Chapter 4.

Non-Confrontational Language

Employing non-confrontational language is vital for promoting constructive conversations. Using "I" statements helps express feelings and thoughts without attributing blame, which can prevent defensive reactions. Instead of saying, "You never communicate," a parent could frame it as, "I feel disconnected when we don't talk often." This shift focuses on the parent's feelings, creating an atmosphere of collaboration rather than conflict. The emphasis is on openness and vulnerability, allowing both parties to share their experiences and emotions candidly.

Clear Boundaries

Boundaries establish a respectful environment, helping both parents and children navigate discussions without escalating tensions. Agreeing on parameters such as how often to communicate or topics to avoid ensures that the conversation remains productive. For instance, a boundary might be avoiding discussions about certain sensitive topics during family gatherings, preventing emotionally charged exchanges. Clear boundaries foster mutual respect and allow each party to feel heard and secure. This structure not only aids in communication but also reinforces a healthy dynamic as the relationship evolves.

Follow-Up Conversations

After initial discussions, parents should proactively reach out to continue the conversation, even if there isn't immediate resolution. Sending a message or planning a coffee meeting reiterates dedication to the process. It shows the child that rebuilding the relationship is a priority and that efforts are sustained beyond a singular discussion. These talks reinforce the commitment to ongoing dialogue, strengthening connection and trust over time. Regular check-ins demonstrate patience, allowing space for both parties to reflect on previous talks and progress collaboratively toward mending the relationship.

The path toward reconciliation is unique for each family, and these tools, while powerful, require consistent application and adaptation. Parents should remember that healing doesn't occur overnight, and setbacks may happen. Patience and perseverance are key.

The Importance of Self-Reflection

Parents must remain mindful of their own emotional needs. Engaging in self-reflection can help them identify any triggers or biases that might affect interactions, fostering a compassionate approach to themselves and their children.

For example, Marcus and his daughter Jane haven't spoken in several months. Although he misses his daughter, Marcus is hurt since Jane decided to stop attending religious services and declared she no longer professes the faith she was raised into. Marcus, a deeply religious man, feels his daughter isn't only rejecting his teachings and family values, but also dismissing him as a father.

Just like him, a parent might find it difficult to discuss certain past events due to deeply ingrained emotions or unresolved conflict. In such instances, acknowledging these feelings internally can prepare them for future discussions, ensuring that their responses remain measured and understanding. Engaging with support groups or therapy can offer additional insights and coping strategies, further equipping them to handle complex emotions with grace and empathy.

After talking to a spiritual advisor, Marcus understands his daughter needs to walk her path, and even when he doesn't agree with all her choices, this doesn't mean he has failed as a parent. On the contrary, he can finally appreciate the strength in Jane that allowed her to make such a difficult decision by herself. Recognizing personal growth areas complements their efforts in communication, contributing to a more harmonious rebuilding process.

Equally important is recognizing that circumstances and willingness to reconcile may vary between family members. While one may be eager to reconnect, the other might need more time. Understanding and respecting this disparity allows relationships to grow at a natural pace, minimizing pressure and potential friction. Encouraging honest discourse about readiness and expectations provides clarity, aligning intentions and creating space for authentic connections to flourish.

Seeking Professional Help

Maybe you and your estranged child aren't ready to fix the relationship all by yourselves, and in that case, it's worth asking for help. Counseling can be a transformative step for families seeking to reconcile with their estranged children. It provides an essential neutral ground where both parents and children are guided through discussions in an unbiased manner by trained therapists. In these sessions, each party is encouraged to express their feelings and perspectives without fear of judgment or backlash.

Through counseling, misunderstandings that may have remained unaddressed for years can finally be brought to light and resolved. By introducing new ways of interacting, families can break free from entrenched patterns of arguments and disagreements (Chae, n.d.). Here are some strategies that work.

Mediation

One of the most effective tools available in this setting is mediation techniques. These methods provide structure and facilitate a collaborative approach to conflict resolution. Mediation encourages both parents and children to voice their needs openly and work together toward finding common ground. It's crucial though to understand that the process of reconciliation isn't quick or easy. Parents and children must both commit genuine effort to the journey of healing. Recognizing that such efforts take time is vital to creating an environment where long-lasting resolutions can emerge.

Find the Right Professional

Selecting the right professional to guide this process is crucial. An experienced therapist who understands family dynamics can significantly enhance the effectiveness of therapy sessions. A good professional not only mediates but also helps build trust and rapport within the family, encouraging individuals to open up and engage genuinely with the process.

To choose wisely, it may be beneficial to research potential counselors' backgrounds and approaches to therapy. Asking questions about their experience with similar family situations can help determine if they are the right fit for your needs. It's important for the family to feel comfortable with the chosen therapist, as this will encourage a more honest and productive dialogue during sessions (Messina, 2023).

A Two-Side Commitment

The commitment required for successful counseling extends beyond attending sessions. It involves a willingness from all involved to actively participate and apply the principles learned during therapy to everyday interactions. This might include practicing communication techniques at home, engaging in exercises aimed at improving mutual understanding, or simply committing to spend more quality time together as a family.

The path to reconciliation requires ongoing effort, patience, and a willingness to embrace change. More than just resolving issues, therapy can promote individual growth and self-awareness, which enhances overall family health.

Final Insights

Family estrangement can be a daunting challenge, but with the right tools, you can manage to rebuild connections between you and your adult children.

- Through effective communication strategies like active listening and non-confrontational language, parents can create a safe space for open dialogue.

- By setting clear boundaries and engaging in follow-up discussions, families can nurture trust and demonstrate a commitment to repairing relationships that have suffered over time.

- Seeking counseling or mediation can be pivotal, offering a neutral environment where families can openly express feelings and address misunderstandings.

- Choosing a qualified therapist who understands family dynamics enhances the effectiveness of these efforts.

- Committing to therapy involves consistent application of learned communication techniques, emphasizing growth both as individuals and as a family unit.

Each family's path to reconciliation will look different, yet these approaches provide a solid foundation for moving forward with care and patience.

On the other hand, sometimes, reconciliation doesn't seem possible, at least not in the short term. Our next chapter will explore strategies on how to support your children despite the distance—both physical and emotional.

Chapter 4:

Supporting Your Child From a Distance

I encountered a woman named Louise—her name changed for confidentiality—who had lost her connection with her son, Rob. Over time, she discovered the painful truth: Rob had been a victim of severe physical abuse at the hands of his father during his childhood. Though Louise insisted she was oblivious to the horrors unfolding within their home and that the abuser had long since vanished, Rob found it impossible to absolve her. To him, she had neglected her duty to safeguard him from harm.

The estrangement weighs heavily on Louise, compounded by the reality of grandchildren she has yet to meet. Despite her deep yearning for reconnection, she recognizes that Rob requires considerable time and space to process his trauma. This journey of healing is personal and cannot be rushed.

Louise understands that attempting to force a reconciliation would likely do more harm than good. She has come to appreciate that true healing must precede any effort to rebuild their relationship. Patience, she realizes, is crucial as Rob navigates the emotional turmoil rooted in his past.

While the distance between them is painful, Louise's empathy allows her to support Rob from afar. She hopes that, in time, he will find the strength to confront his past and perhaps one day extend a hand toward rebuilding their bond. Louise's love remains steadfast, illuminating her path as she waits for the day they might reconnect.

Your situation may or may not be as drastic as Louise's. In any case, supporting your child from a distance presents a unique set of challenges that many parents find themselves navigating as their children grow older and gain independence—by the way, this equally applies to families who haven't suffered from estrangement!

In this chapter, we'll explore the reality of supporting a child from afar, highlighting the importance of listening to understand rather than to respond. Understanding personal boundaries is also a key focus. Additionally, we discuss identifying potential triggers in communication that may lead to conflict, providing strategies for approaching sensitive topics with care.

The strategies we'll explore aren't just meant to amend a broken relationship, but to prevent family estrangement in the first place, or new conflict after any party attempts a reconciliation. Particularly in the case of family estrangement, by emphasizing empathy and patience, parents can create an environment where their child feels comfortable reaching out for guidance when needed, without feeling overwhelmed or pushed.

Reaching Out to Your Estranged Child

If you are feeling heartbroken and discouraged for losing touch with your adult child, stay hopeful. Cling to the thought that forgiveness is possible. It may help you to know that, according to research from the Newport Institute, 8 out of 10 cases of estrangement involving mothers, and almost 7 out of 10 involving fathers, end up in some sort of reconciliation (*Parental Estrangement*, 2024).

No matter who started the estrangement, the ball is in the parents' court when it comes to reaching out. According to Dr. Joshua Coleman, psychologist and author, whenever a reconciliation takes place, the parent needs to "at least be willing to look at their own part in why the adult child has created such a powerful form of distance" (Anderson, 2014). So even if you feel you have done nothing wrong, it is still up to you—to some point—to reach out to your child. How can you attempt it without seemingly breaking your adult child's boundaries and disrespecting their choice?

- Assess your expectations—and let them go. If your motivation is to fix a broken relationship, you're more likely to be disappointed. Instead, try to reconnect to understand the causes behind your child's decision.

- Respect your adult child's boundaries. If they've made clear they don't want to see you, bumping into them in their workplace or trying to see your grandkids when they go out of school is likely to drive your adult child further away.

- Write them a letter. Reaching out by letter or email allows your child to process their emotions, leaving them time to respond without pressuring them for a face-to-face encounter.

- Apologize, but don't expect immediate forgiveness. It may take a lot of patience and perseverance from your side.

- Be unconditional when you try to reconnect. Now is not the time to address your feelings of loneliness and despair because of the estrangement, much less to criticize or question your child's motivations.

But what if, after sending letters, touching texts, and voice messages, your children still refuse to acknowledge your attempts to reconnect? Is there a moment you should stop trying and move on? According to Dr. Coleman, although this is hard, allowing your child the distance they request can be the most loving parental action for the time being: "If things are so inflamed that you're getting threatened with restraining orders or your gifts are being sent back, then they're too inflamed for progress to be made by reaching out" (2020). In that case, you can always end your attempts by leaving the door open, telling them in one last message that you love and respect them, and they can always reach out if they need you.

Understanding Their Perspective and Needs

In the complex dance of parenting, finding ways to support your children without overstepping can be challenging. If you and your adult child have gone through a period of estrangement, and you are slowly reconnecting, understanding their thoughts and feelings is crucial for fostering empathy and building a stronger relationship.

Revisiting the Importance of Active Listening

As mentioned in Chapter 3, active listening requires parents to engage in conversations with their children without judgment. This means putting aside preconceived notions or solutions and allowing children to express themselves freely. Parents create a safe space for their children to reveal deeper emotions and concerns they might otherwise keep hidden. For instance, an estranged adult child may refer to a past episode that the parent thinks wasn't such a big deal, and in that case, their child may need an empathetic ear to understand why it affected them emotionally.

By truly listening, parents gain insight into these underlying issues, facilitating a supportive environment where children feel heard and valued. According to *The Center for Parenting Education* (2012), employing this technique is pivotal—listening first helps empower children to articulate their feelings and, eventually, solve their own problems.

Beyond listening, seeking clarity through open-ended questions can profoundly impact understanding your adult child's perspective. Instead of asking yes-or-no questions like, "Did I do something wrong?" try asking, "If given the chance, what would you change about our history together?" Such questions encourage your adult child to elaborate on their experiences and explore their feelings more deeply.

This approach enhances mutual understanding by inviting detailed responses, offering parents a clearer window into their adult child's personal recollection of events. Through this method, parents are not merely extracting information but establishing an environment where their children feel comfortable expressing themselves, and aiding in reducing misunderstandings.

Honoring Boundaries

Recognizing personal boundaries is another critical aspect of supporting adult children from a distance. Each person has distinct comfort levels regarding privacy and sharing personal information. Parents need to acknowledge and respect these boundaries, which encourages healthy interactions and prevents overwhelming the child.

This is particularly important when there was an estrangement. For example, your adult child may finally agree on emails or voicemails, but not feel ready for a face-to-face meeting, and pushing them could result in resistance or even withdrawal. Respecting these boundaries demonstrates trust and shows that parents honor their adult child's autonomy and need for space.

If this is the case, always thank your child for agreeing on whatever contact they are okay with, and leave the door open for future possibilities of reconnection: "I'm glad you're responding to my emails. It makes me happy to get news from you. Remember we can meet whenever you are ready for it." Over time, as trust builds, your adult child may become more willing to share experiences and establish a closer relationship once more.

Recognizing and Understanding Triggers

Just like active listening and boundaries, understanding triggers is equally important in maintaining harmonious relationships. Parents must recognize situations or topics that provoke negative responses in their adult children. For instance, if your child cut you off because you two disagreed on certain values or decisions, bringing up the topic may trigger stress or defiance. Identifying these triggers allows parents to navigate conversations more thoughtfully, avoiding potential conflict. By being mindful of what subjects might evoke strong reactions, parents can approach discussions with greater sensitivity and patience. This proactive strategy helps maintain open lines of communication, ensuring conversations remain constructive rather than confrontational.

Moreover, addressing and resolving these issues together creates a collaborative atmosphere where adult children don't feel attacked or misunderstood. They learn to communicate their needs effectively, while parents provide a supportive backdrop for problem-solving, ultimately enhancing the emotional connection between parent and child.

Balancing Support Without Overstepping Boundaries

Supporting your child from a distance can be challenging, yet it's crucial to find the balance between offering support and respecting their autonomy. In the end, if your adult child decided to cut ties with the family, it is still an adult decision—one you disagree with, but nonetheless should respect.

Set Norms

As you work toward rebuilding the relationship, remember that establishing communication norms with your child is an essential first step. By setting agreements on how and when to communicate, both parties can manage expectations and respect each other's time. Such norms reduce misunderstandings and ensure that interactions are productive rather than intrusive. These agreements might involve scheduling regular phone calls or determining the best times for messaging. It's vital to consider factors such as time zones if you're separated by distance. Open dialogue about these norms can prevent potential conflicts.

Be Available, Don't Impose Your Help

Subtlety in offering help can make a significant difference in supporting your child. Let's take Johanna and her daughter Mindy, who has a three-year-old son named Luke. For a whole year, they became estranged because Mindy disagreed on how Johanna looked after Luke. She felt her mother didn't respect her indications and constantly criticized her parenting style. Eventually, Mindy and Johanna reconnected, but the daughter is still sensitive to criticism—albeit overwhelmed by trying to balance being a mom and working full time.

Rather than imposing assistance, Johanna should suggest opportunities where Mindy might feel empowered. For example, she could say, "I know you've been busy; let me know if you need any help," instead of directly offering unsolicited advice or aid. This approach respects Mindy's capability to manage her challenges while letting her know Mom is available when needed. Observing their comfort levels is also key—being attentive to cues on whether they seem overwhelmed or managing well will guide your interactions appropriately.

Assess Yourself

Regularly practicing self-reflection is a critical component in ensuring you remain supportive while respecting your adult child's independence and don't push them back. Reflect on your actions and assess whether they align with your child's needs and desires. This involves being honest with yourself about your motivations—are you offering advice out of habit, or because it would genuinely benefit your child? Understanding your emotional responses is important, especially when feeling rejected or excluded. Seek feedback from your adult child to better understand their perspective and adjust your approach accordingly.

Concluding Thoughts

Throughout this chapter, we've explored the delicate balance between providing support and respecting your adult child's independence, especially when you are trying to rebuild the relationship.

- By focusing on active listening, parents can create a nurturing environment where children feel both understood and valued.

- Engaging in open-ended conversations encourages children to express themselves more fully, allowing for deeper mutual understanding.

- Recognizing and respecting your child's boundaries helps establish trust and strengthens the parent-child relationship.

- It's important for parents to practice self-reflection, ensuring that their actions align with their child's needs and desires.

As you continue to embrace these strategies, remember to maintain an open dialogue, offering subtle guidance while honoring your adult child's autonomy. Together, these efforts contribute to a healthy, respectful relationship that moves on from past conflict and faces a brighter future.

While you keep reconnection as your goal, you must accept to live with the reality of estrangement at the same time. Our last chapter will teach you about optimism and resilience.

Chapter 5:

Staying Resilient and Hopeful

Maintaining a positive attitude when facing family estrangement is an intricate dance between cultivating personal strength and harboring optimism for reconciliation. When faced with the pain of estrangement from an adult child, it's easy to feel lost and uncertain about what the future holds. Such a challenging experience can test the very core of one's emotional and mental framework, leaving individuals grappling with feelings of despair and confusion. However, resilience doesn't mean the absence of adversity; rather, it involves enduring tough times with the belief that brighter days lie ahead. By focusing on developing a resilient mindset, parents not only brace themselves against the emotional storms but also keep the hope of eventual reunion alive.

In this chapter, we delve into various strategies designed to bolster resilience and foster hope during such trying times. Hopefully, these tips will manage to provide you with the tools needed to not just survive, but thrive in the face of familial estrangement, holding onto the hope that healing remains possible.

Building a Support Network

Engaging with a supportive community is crucial for navigating the emotional turmoil of estrangement. For many parents facing separation from their adult children, the sense of isolation can be overwhelming. Surrounding yourself with friends and family who understand your situation not only alleviates this loneliness but also provides diverse perspectives that may shed new light on your circumstances. Such personal connections invite shared experiences and empathy, offering mental and emotional relief.

Support Groups

Joining support groups specifically designed for parents dealing with estrangement can be transformative. These groups provide an invaluable space where individuals can come together to share their stories and gain collective wisdom. Participants often report how hearing others' experiences normalizes their own feelings of loss and validates emotions they might have struggled to articulate. Support groups cultivate a community spirit where members find solidarity in knowing they are not alone, which ultimately helps in rebuilding hope and resilience. The insights gained from such interactions can shift one's perspective and encourage a more proactive approach to coping with the estrangement.

Online Communities

In our digital age, online communities offer a unique platform to connect with individuals worldwide who are experiencing similar situations. These communities thrive on anonymity and a shared commitment to mutual support. Engaging with these forums can help mitigate feelings of hopelessness by offering constant engagement and feedback from peers who truly understand your plight.

Friends You Trust

It's important to actively seek out trusted friends who have undergone similar experiences with estrangement. Their firsthand insights can offer validation and reassurance during challenging times. Consulting someone who has navigated this difficult journey can provide a new perspective on effective coping mechanisms. Personal conversations with such friends create opportunities to express emotions tied to estrangement, allowing for a cathartic release while receiving practical advice on managing these intense feelings. Their stories of resilience can inspire hope by demonstrating that forward movement is possible, even when reconciliation seems uncertain or far off.

To ensure that engaging with these communities is genuinely helpful, it's vital to choose connections wisely. Select friends and family members who show genuine understanding and empathy toward your experience. This requires an honest evaluation of your current relationships and recognizing those who truly listen without judgment. It might be beneficial to establish boundaries regarding what is shared, ensuring discussions remain constructive and focused on healing rather than dwelling on past hurts.

Each estrangement situation is unique, and what worked for one person might not necessarily work for another. Approach these dialogues with an open mind, ready to absorb various strategies and viewpoints, which can then be adapted to suit your personal context.

Exploring Self-Help Strategies and Resources

In the difficult journey of navigating estrangement from an adult child, building emotional resilience becomes a cornerstone for maintaining hope and personal stability. Parents who experience such life-altering situations often find themselves in uncharted territories of emotional distress and uncertainty. It is during these times that practical self-help strategies can act as guiding lights, carving paths toward inner peace and strength. Let's explore some key approaches.

Mindfulness

Practicing mindfulness and meditation is a vital tool for grounding oneself amidst emotional turmoil. When relationships become strained or severed, parents might feel untethered, overwhelmed by cascading thoughts and emotions. Mindfulness helps anchor the mind to the present moment, reducing anxiety and bringing a sense of calm and clarity. Through meditation, one learns to observe thoughts without judgment, understanding them as transient rather than defining. Regular practice fosters a resilient mindset, enabling individuals to respond thoughtfully rather than react impulsively (Stang, 2024). Try starting with just five minutes a day, focusing on breathing or listening to guided meditations.

Keep a Journal

Alongside mindfulness, keeping a journal is a powerful means of processing emotional experiences. The act of writing allows parents to articulate and navigate their feelings concerning estrangement. Journaling provides a space to vent frustrations, capture fleeting thoughts, or express deep-seated fears and hopes. This exercise serves as a cathartic release, allowing complex emotions to be unraveled and understood in a safe environment. Over time, recurring patterns or insights may emerge, offering clarity and guiding decisions regarding the future of familial relationships. A simple guideline to follow could be setting aside a few minutes each evening to jot down daily reflections or notable events.

Take Up a Hobby

Engaging in new hobbies is another effective strategy to inspire joy and provide distraction from the pain of estrangement. Discovering activities that spark interest can help parents reconnect with aspects of their identity beyond their role within the family. Whether it's painting, gardening, learning a musical instrument, or any creative pursuit, new hobbies are opportunities to channel energy into constructive outlets. Not only do they serve as distractions, but they can also reignite passions and remind individuals of their latent potential and interests. Such engagements are valuable reminders that life holds various facets worth exploring and celebrating regardless of personal hardships.

Read

Reading self-help literature focused on coping with estrangement offers knowledge and empowerment through shared stories and professional insights. Books that delve into similar experiences provide solace in knowing others have navigated comparable paths, offering strategies that worked in diverse circumstances (Suri & Mohan, 2024). Authors often share tools and exercises aimed at fostering resilience and nurturing self-understanding. This literature not only imparts practical advice but also reinforces the notion that healing and growth remain possible despite current adversities. As parents immerse themselves in these narratives, they may find newfound perspectives and hope, vital companions in their journey of personal recovery.

Insights and Implications

In the face of estrangement, building a support network becomes a lifeline of both understanding and strength.

- Surround yourself with friends, family, and like-minded individuals who truly empathize with your situation to alleviate feelings of isolation.

- Participating in support groups or engaging with online communities tailored to parents dealing with estrangement can bring a sense of belonging and shared experience.

- The importance of selecting supportive and empathetic companions cannot be overstated, as this choice greatly affects your journey toward resilience and hope.

Alongside these community connections, nurturing personal resilience through self-help strategies is key. Practices such as mindfulness, journaling, and exploring new hobbies can aid in grounding your emotions and rediscovering joy outside the confines of familial roles. Engaging with self-help literature also adds valuable perspectives and guidance. Each tool contributes uniquely to the healing process, reminding you that while reconciliation may not be immediate, it is the strength and hope cultivated within yourself and your community that empower you to navigate this challenging path. In these actions and insights, the seeds of healing are planted, offering a path forward filled with potential for growth and understanding.

Conclusion

As we stand together at the crossroads of understanding and reconciliation, it is essential to embrace the multifaceted nature of estrangement. This journey has revealed that the paths leading to family separations are often tangled with the threads of personal choices and broader societal narratives. From media portrayals to shifting generational values, these outside influences weave into the intimate fabric of family life, creating scenarios that can push adult children and parents apart. Understanding this complexity allows the ability to step back, view the whole picture, and grasp the nuances without jumping to conclusions. When parents recognize that their experience is shaped by a myriad of factors, they open themselves up to a deeper empathy—both for themselves and their estranged children.

But with understanding must come action, and there is perhaps no greater tool in bridging divides than communication. Here, we underscore the transformative power of respectful dialogue. The approach taken within each conversation can lay the foundation for either healing or further conflict. Effective communication is about more than speaking; it's rooted in active listening—a practice where each party truly hears and acknowledges the other's perspective. It demands that language remain free from confrontation, that boundaries be honored, and that the aim is not to win an argument but to share experiences and emotions honestly. In creating these safer spaces, parents and children alike find the opportunity to lower defenses, potentially paving the path toward healing wounds that might have seemed impossible to mend.

Yet, even with improved understanding and communication, the journey through estrangement should not be walked alone. Establishing a strong support system is vital. Whether it is through friends who have stood by for years, fellow parents experiencing similar struggles, professional counselors, or community support groups, these connections provide a lifeline. They offer validation in moments of self-doubt and comfort on days when isolation feels overwhelming.

Amidst all these efforts, fostering resilience and nurturing hope are the guiding lights that keep us moving forward. Estrangement tests emotional strength in profound ways, yet within every challenge lies the seed of resilience. By focusing on self-care and personal well-being, parents can empower themselves to face emotional turbulence with grace. Self-care isn't a luxury reserved for better days; it's a crucial commitment to oneself. Activities such as mindfulness, meditation, or even leisure hobbies help maintain a balanced mental state while reinforcing self-worth. Hope, like a resilient tether, binds us to the possibility of reconciliation. Even if past attempts have faltered, maintaining hope invites new opportunities and potential beginnings, offering a lens through which future relationships can flourish.

As we draw these reflections to a close, I want to thank you. To the parents bravely seeking understanding amidst heartache, thank you for allowing this book to be part of your journey. To mental health professionals dedicated to supporting families grappling with estrangement, your work is invaluable, and your empathy makes a world of difference. We end with a request: If this exploration has resonated with you and offered solace or a sense of direction, please consider sharing your thoughts in a review. Your feedback not only assists other readers in discovering these insights but also contributes to the broader conversation surrounding family dynamics and healing.

Families, no matter how fragmented, hold the inherent potential for change and growth. As you continue to navigate your unique situation, remember that each day presents a new opportunity to understand, communicate, connect, and heal. Though the journey may be long and hard, each step is meaningful, and every effort toward reconciliation, no matter how small, is worthwhile.

References

Anderson, J. (2014). *Estranged: What to do when your adult child wants nothing to do with you.* Lifewise By Dr. Jan. https://www.drjananderson.com/blog/estranged-what-to-do-when-your-adult-child-wants-nothing-to-do-with-you

Brindle, K. C. (2024, May 28). *Community support of someone who is estranged.* Croswaite Counseling PLLC. https://croswaitecounselingpllc.com/blog/2024/5/28/community-support-of-someone-who-is-estranged

Brooks, S. K., & Greenberg, N. (2020, August 17). *Psychological impact of being wrongfully accused of criminal offences: a systematic literature review.* Medicine, Science and the Law. https://www.ncbi.nlm.nih.gov/pmc/articles/PMC7838333/

Burford, M. (2024, May 17). *Coping with grief and loss: 6 tips for healing.* Oak Street Health. https://www.oakstreethealth.com/coping-with-grief-and-loss-6-tips-for-healing-1782782

Carlson, M. (2015, April 20). *Active Listening: How to master the skill that will make you a more effective parent.* A Fine Parent. https://afineparent.com/emotional-intelligence/active-listening.html

Catchings, C. V. (2025, February 21). *Healing estranged relationships with your adult children.* Talkspace. https://www.talkspace.com/blog/estranged-adult-children/

The Center for Parenting Education. (2012). *The skill of listening.* https://centerforparentingeducation.org/library-of-articles/healthy-communication/the-skill-of-listening/

Chae, C. (n.d.). *Healthy family dynamics: The role of therapy.* Abundance Therapy Center. https://www.abundancetherapycenter.com/blog/healthy-family-dynamics-the-role-of-therapy

Coleman, J. (2020, May 6). *Why should you stop trying with your estranged adult child?* Psychology Today. https://www.psychologytoday.com/intl/blog/the-rules-of-estrangement/202005/why-should-you-stop-trying-with-your-estranged-adult-child

Coping with family estrangement: How to heal and move forward. (2024). Inner Strength Therapy. https://innerstrengththerapyllc.com/coping-with-family-estrangement-how-to-heal-and-move-forward

Dashnaw, D. (2024, June 24). *Should I keep reaching out to my estranged adult child?* Daniel Dashnaw Couples Therapy. https://danieldashnawcouplestherapy.com/blog/should-i-keep-reaching-out-to-my-estranged-adult-child

Dean, J. (2020, September 10). *Pillemer: Family estrangement a problem 'hiding in plain sight.'* Cornell Chronicle. https://news.cornell.edu/stories/2020/09/pillemer-family-estrangement-problem-hiding-plain-sight

Ergenzinger, E. (2022, May 4). *Mourning the living: Mental illness and family estrangement.* Psychology Today. https://www.psychologytoday.com/us/blog/night-sweats-and-delusions-of-grandeur/202205/mourning-the-living-mental-illness-and-family

Henkelman, P. (2024). *Decoding parental estrangement: Understanding the root causes*. Pamela Henkelman. https://www.pamelahenkelman.com/articles/decoding-parental-estrangement-understanding-the-root-causes

Lis, L. (2022, March 31). *Growing up with a narcissistic mother.* Psychology Today. https://www.psychologytoday.com/intl/blog/the-shameless-psychiatrist/202203/growing-narcissistic-mother

Livingston, T. (2024, September 4). *Understanding & coping with estrangement: Define estranged and steps to reconcile.* BlueNotary Online Notarization. https://bluenotary.us/define-estranged/

McGregor, S. (2024, May 22). *My adult child is a narcissist: Is it my fault?* Done With the Crying. https://www.rejectedparents.net/my-adult-child-is-a-narcissist-is-it-my-fault/

Messina, D. M. (2023, October 9). *Family counseling: Strengthening bonds & resolving conflicts.* Dr. Messina & Associates. https://drmessina.com/family-counseling-strengthening-bonds-resolving-conflicts/

Morin, M. (2023, July 5). *Seven keys to dealing with estranged adult-children with mental illness.* Morin Holistic Therapy. https://morinholistictherapy.com/seven-keys-to-dealing-with-estranged-adult-children-with-mental-illness/

Parental estrangement: Can the family heal after adult children divorce their parents? (2024). Newport Institute. https://www.newportinstitute.com/resources/mental-health/parental-estrangement/

Procentese F, Gatti F, Di Napoli I. *Families and social media use: The role of parents' perceptions about social media impact on family systems in the relationship between family collective efficacy and open communication.* Int J Environ Res Public Health. 2019 Dec 9;16(24):5006. doi: 10.3390/ijerph16245006. PMID: 31835396; PMCID: PMC6950110.

Stang, H. (2024, December 4). *Cope with family estrangement during the holidays: Mindful Tips for Emotional Well-Being.* Mindfulness & Grief Support for Loss with Author Heather Stang. https://heatherstang.com/family-estrangement-during-the-holiday/

Streep, P. (2023, May 20). *No, parent-child estrangement isn't just a fad.* Psychology Today. https://www.psychologytoday.com/us/blog/tech-support/202305/no-adult-childparent-estrangement-isnt-a-fad

Suri, R.K. & Mohan, M. (2024). *Healing from family estrangement.* TalktoAngel. https://www.talktoangel.com/blog/healing-from-family-estrangement

Trepany, P. (2024, January 23). *Narcissists wreak havoc on their parents' lives. But cutting them off can feel impossible.* USA Today. https://www.usatoday.com/story/life/health-wellness/2024/01/23/narcissists-children-parents-how-to-cope/72316068007/

Uncovering the nightmare: When you're falsely accused of a crime. (2023, December 3). Henry & Beaver. https://henrybeaver.com/uncovering-the-nightmare-when-youre-falsely-accused-of-a-crime/

Printed in Great Britain
by Amazon